THE MIDWIFE

Susan Cohen

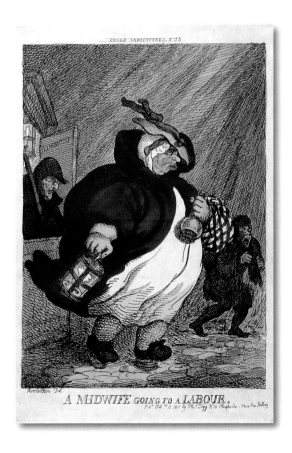

A MIDWIFE GOING TO A LABOUR

Published in Great Britain in 2016 by Shire Publications Ltd (part of Bloomsbury Publishing Plc), PO Box 883, Oxford, OX1 9PL, UK.

PO Box 3985, New York, NY 10185-3985, USA.

E-mail: shire@shirebooks.co.uk
www.shirebooks.co.uk

A CIP catalogue record for this book is available from the British Library.

Shire Library no. 821.   ISBN-13: 978 0 74781 507 5

PDF e-book ISBN: 978 1 78442 094 9

ePub ISBN: 978 1 78442 093 2

Susan Cohen has asserted her right under the Copyright, Designs and Patents Act, 1988, to be identified as the author of this book.

Typeset in Garamond Pro and Gill Sans.

Printed in China through World Print Ltd.

16 17 18 19 20   10 9 8 7 6 5 4 3 2 1

COVER IMAGE
A midwife weighs a baby while visiting a family at home, March 1965. (Topfoto)

TITLE PAGE IMAGE
Thomas Rowlandson's caricature, about 1811, represents a stereotypical view of midwives in the early nineteenth century as blowsy, obese, ignorant and prone to drink – one verse about midwives described them as 'Taking snuff, drinking gin and tea, and the midwife's half-crown fee.'

CONTENTS PAGE IMAGE
A mother and her newborn baby going home from hospital, c. 1950s.

ACKNOWLEDGEMENTS
A special thank you to Penny Hutchins for her invaluable assistance with providing images from the Royal College of Midwives collection at the Royal College of Obstetricians and Gynaecologists. Also, thanks to Nicky Leap and Billie Hunter for permission to include quotes from The Midwife's Tale, and to Lindsay Reid for allowing me to quote from Scottish Midwives.

Photograph acknowledgements can be found on page 63.

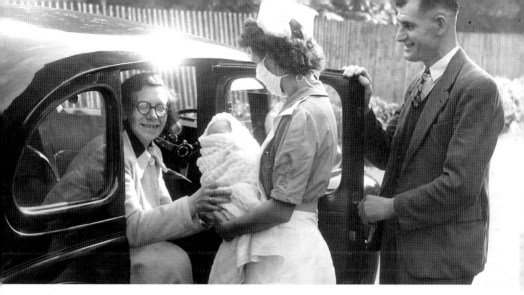

CONTENTS

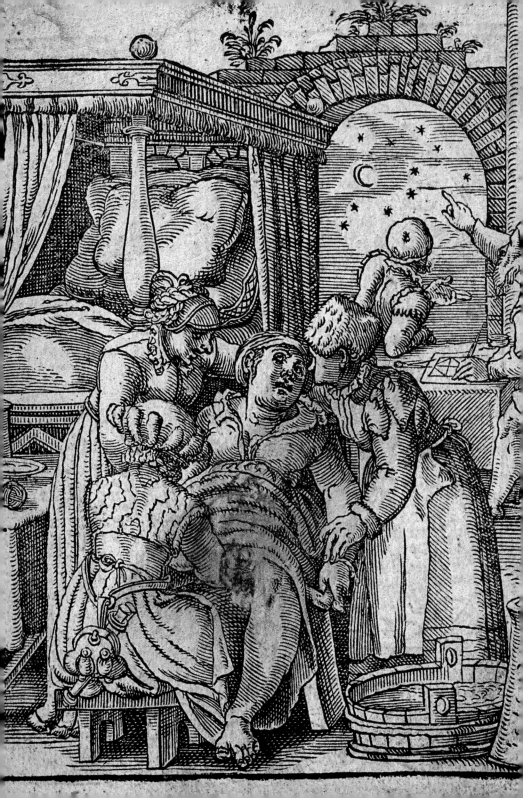

THE EARLY DAYS

THE ROLE OF the midwife, attending to and assisting women in childbirth, has been recorded since time immemorial, but the traditionally female practice was unregulated, and was not officially recognised as a profession in Britain until the Midwives Act was passed in England and Wales in July 1902. This was undoubtedly a turning point, but was just the beginning of a long process, fraught with difficulties and debate, during which midwifery developed to become the highly skilled branch of nursing, open to men and women, which is recognisable today.

For centuries, practitioners were a motley crew, ranging from the handywoman, epitomised in the nineteenth century by Charles Dickens' character, Sairy Gamp, to the careful, knowledgeable and empathetic midwife. Handywomen, who typically acted as midwife, monthly nurse and the layer-out of the dead, were commonly unhygienic, illiterate and frequently dangerous, but were all that was available to poor women. The best and the safest birth attendants, engaged by the more discerning and educated in society, learnt their craft from their mothers or an elder, served lengthy apprenticeships and, in turn, passed their knowledge onto the next generation. Flora Thompson's fictional rural midwife, old Mrs Quinton, in *Lark Rise to Candleford*, was one such woman, who recognised a rare crisis and the need to call the doctor. She took pride in her work and was valued by the local doctor, who appreciated the important role she played in the community.

Opposite:
A seated woman giving birth aided by a midwife and two other attendants. In the background, two men are looking at the stars and plotting a horoscope. Woodcut, about 1583.

Below: This caricature by Isaac Cruikshank, about 1793, depicts the man-midwife as a split figure – half male, half female.

Below right: Mrs Sarah Stone's textbook, *A Complete Practice of Midwifery* (1737), was intended for 'all female practitioners in an art so important to the lives and well-being of the sex.'

Childbirth was viewed as a natural process, with ordinary married women or widows acting as midwives or handywomen. They helped their neighbours give birth and provided practical help with childcare and domestic tasks; in return they earned a modest livelihood. Most midwives were, like their patients, educationally disadvantaged. Even if they were literate, as women they were denied the opportunity to learn anatomy, attend lectures or read the specialist books traditionally written in Latin and Greek. Mrs Jane Sharp was one of the earliest midwives to put her wealth of experience to practical use by publishing the first English textbook for midwives in 1671: *The Midwives Book*, which was also aimed at mothers and fathers, and provided advice on conception, pregnancy, the birth itself and postnatal care, along with anatomical illustrations and descriptions of difficult births. Another midwife, Mrs Sarah Stone of Taunton, whose book *A Complete Practice of Midwifery* followed in 1737,

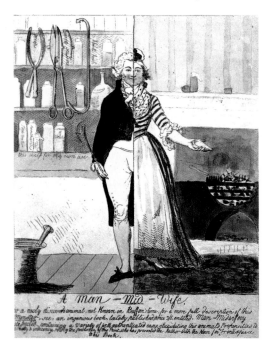

A man – mid – wife.

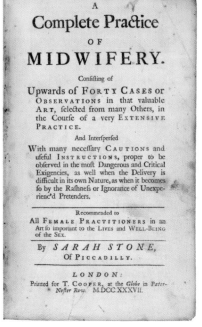

A

Complete Practice

OF

MIDWIFERY.

Confifting of

Upwards of FORTY CASES or OBSERVATIONS in that valuable ART, felected from many Others, in the Courfe of a very EXTENSIVE PRACTICE.

And Interfperfed

With many neceffary CAUTIONS and ufeful INSTRUCTIONS, proper to be obferved in the moft Dangerous and Critical Exigencies, as well when the Delivery is difficult in its own Nature, as when it becomes fo by the Rafhnefs or Ignorance of Unexperienc'd Pretenders.

Recommended to

All FEMALE PRACTITIONERS in an Art fo important to the LIVES and WELL-BEING of the SEX.

By SARAH STONE, Of PICCADILLY.

LONDON:

Printed for T. COOPER, at the *Globe* in Pater-Nofter Row. M.DCC.XXXVII.

was intended to 'ignite the confidence of even midwives of the lowest capacity' so they could 'deliver their women, without calling in, or sending for, a Man, in every little seeming difficulty.'

The man-midwife was not new, but was gaining a foothold in upper-class circles from the 1700s, on the basis that he had 'superior' knowledge. This received wisdom was clearly not always the case for, as Mrs Stone pointed out, some had very dubious qualifications, including the pork butcher who gave up stuffing sausages to deliver babies, mainly because it was a lucrative business.

These men frequently applied the recently introduced obstetric forceps, which most midwives would not use for fear of the damage and danger they caused mothers and babies. Mrs Stone found the instruments of 'very little use', and reported using them only four times in her life, then declared 'I am certain, where twenty women are delivered

Forceps, about 1740–60. Forceps were first described by Edmund Chapman (died 1738) in his *Treatise on the Improvement of Midwifery* (1733). The steel blades of William Smellie's forceps were covered with leather, and were greased with hog's lard before insertion.

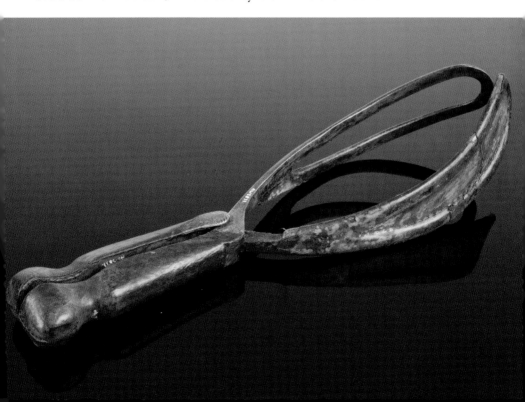

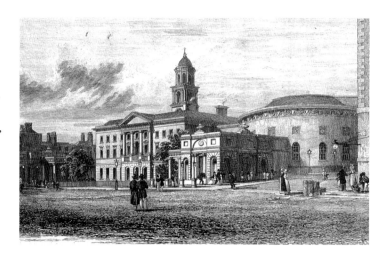

An etching of the Rotunda and Lying-In Hospital, Dublin, Ireland, 1821. Dr Bartholomew Mosse, surgeon and man-midwife, founded the original Dublin Lying-in Hospital in 1745 as a maternity training hospital, the first of its kind. His aim was for every county in Ireland to have a trained midwife.

with instruments (which is now become a common practice) that nineteen of them might be delivered without, if not the twentieth.'

The encroachment of man-midwives had financial implications, even in a relatively small town such as Sheffield. In 1787 there were thirteen surgeon/man-midwives advertising their services, leaving the local midwives with only the very poorest patients to attend. The establishment of more midwifery training courses for men, especially in London, only exacerbated the situation. Amongst the most prestigious were those run by William Smellie, whose book, *A Treatise of the Theory and Practice of Midwifery*, published in 1752, became the foundation of modern midwifery and obstetrics.

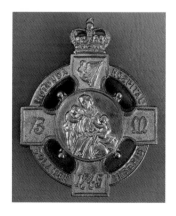

An early badge from the Rotunda hospital. The Dublin Lying-in Hospital moved in 1757, and became known as 'The Rotunda'.

Midwives and handy-women were generally of the same social class as the women they birthed, and were mostly viewed with affection, and admired for the way they did their job. Mrs Heron, whose mother relied upon Martha Blezzard to deliver her eleven children in the late 1800s, remembered her described as 'one of the good old midwives … an ordinary woman with a white apron on … she wasn't certified or anything and it was only a few shillings for a confinement.' Another of her clients remembered her 'as a very nice person' who worked day and night. Martha, or 'Missus' as she was known, used to 'deal with the lot. Then the neighbours used to be around getting hot water. Martha used to get them organised.'

Midwives were strict about a mother staying in bed for up to ten days after childbirth, and it was a practice that was surrounded by superstition. Mrs Drake, born in 1899, related how midwives 'wouldn't let you get up because they said your bones, the backbone, where the child is, they have to knit together.' Another old wives' tale that persisted warned that 'if a mother put her feet on the floor before the ten days were past, she would drop down dead.' Whilst there were genuine concerns about a new mother's recovery, in truth the lying-in period gave her an unprecedented opportunity to rest.

Advertisements such as this one for patented baby milk, about 1880–90, stressed the value of such products as a substitute for breast milk.

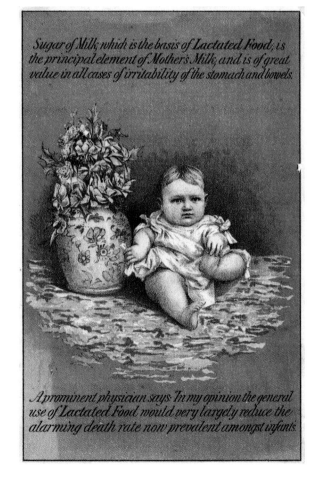

Sugar of Milk, which is the basis of Lactated Food, is the principal element of Mother's Milk, and is of great value in all cases of irritability of the stomach and bowels.

A prominent physician says: 'In my opinion the general use of Lactated Food would very largely reduce the alarming death rate now prevalent amongst infants.'

Pages from an accouchement book listing women attended and babies delivered, about 1889.

An opportunity for midwives to better themselves came in 1872, when the all-male Obstetrical Society of London finally succumbed to pressure from some female campaigners and introduced a diploma, by examination, for women. However, when Miss Sophia Jex-Blake (1840–1912) and two friends, all with impeccable medical and midwifery credentials, were accepted as candidates in 1876, they had a rude awakening, for the three male examiners suddenly refused to conduct the exam and abruptly resigned. This only hardened the resolve of a small band of philanthropic, well-connected women who determined to drive out the uneducated handywomen and get midwifery licensed and regulated.

An example of an early Obstetrical Society of London certificate.

They envisaged the new midwife to be 'a power for good in every home she enters', but she needed training, and before long these enterprising women had established the Midwives' Institute and had set about organising courses of lectures given by doctors and other staff from the London Hospital. Another important initiative was the founding, in 1887, of the institute's journal, *Nursing Notes*, by Rosalind Paget (1855–1948). A trained nurse and newly qualified midwife, Paget financed the establishment of the monthly publication, which campaigned for the professionalisation of midwifery.

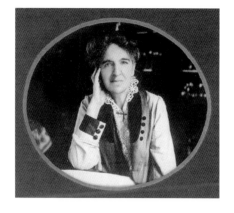

Rosalind Paget gained her Obstetrical Society of London diploma in 1885.

Below: The first members room at the Midwives Institute HQ in London, 1890. By 1984 it had more facilities, including a lecture theatre and smoking room.

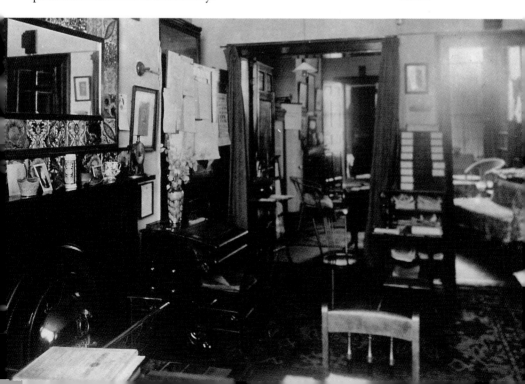

A NEW ERA DAWNS

As the twentieth century dawned, there were still plenty of uncertified handywomen like Martha Blezzard delivering babies, just as they had for generations. But their days were numbered with the passing of the Midwives Act in England and Wales in July 1902. The midwife of the future was to be a trained and enrolled professional, who followed the rules and regulations set out by the newly established Central Midwives Board (CMB), under the chairmanship of Francis Champneys.

The doctors were kept happy as the Act reinforced their monopoly on delivering any case that was not strictly 'normal', therefore protecting their income and professional status. Meanwhile, up until 1905, *bona fides,* those women who could provide sound character references and had at least a year's experience, were automatically eligible to be included on the new Midwives Roll, a measure taken to avoid a sudden national shortage of midwives. These *bona fide* midwives represented nearly half of the 22,308 women listed on 1 April 1905, far more than anticipated, and it was not long before the nursing press were reporting cases of incompetence and other breaches of CMB rules. Drunkenness was a common charge, exemplified by the case of Emma Jones, who was found

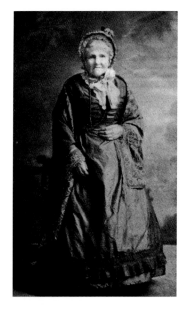

Mrs Rodbard was a *bona fide* midwife who was in practice for forty years. She was seventy-five when this picture was taken in November 1921.

lying in the mother's garden, intoxicated and incapable, and women in such cases could expect to be severely reprimanded and their practice curtailed, or be struck off the official roll.

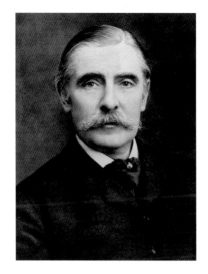

Francis Champneys was chairman of the London Obstetrical Society examining board in 1890, and became president in 1895. He was instrumental in getting the Midwives Act through Parliament.

The aspiring midwife was now faced with a short training course and exams, both of which were a huge stumbling block for all but the best educated and well-off. Mrs Layton, an experienced handywoman, was persuaded to sit the new exam, but she could not afford the fees which ranged from £30 to £50, nor be away from home for three months while she trained. Instead she made do with tuition offered by some local doctors, but she, and about 130 other candidates, failed the exam, and she felt so humiliated that she refused to retake. Other women, including Yiddish-speaking Jewish midwives in East London had to overcome the language obstacles, while the use of Latin medical terms in the exam paper restricted access to all but the educated middle classes.

Initiatives sprang up to train these disadvantaged women, including the Association for Promoting the Training and Supply of Midwives. They opened

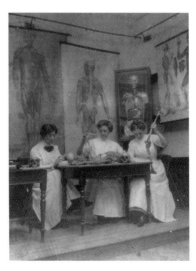

Three midwives learning about anatomy, about 1900.

At this particular Central Midwives Board examination sitting in June 1906, there were 376 candidates, of whom 300 passed. On enquiry, 190 said they intended to practise, ninety-four did not, nine were doubtful and seven did not respond.

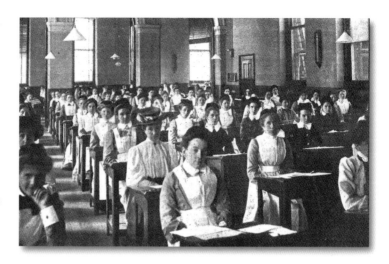

a training school in conjunction with Plaistow Maternity Charity, London and also sponsored training vacancies at several hospitals in London, Glasgow and Cheltenham. Another organization, the Rural Midwives' Association, had successfully sent 136 women for training by 1907, with one hundred of them working across twenty-two counties. Meanwhile, the Midwives' Institute planned three-month-long courses of twice-weekly lectures for pupil midwives, as well as postgraduate lectures for midwives who were training pupils in the district.

The best midwives were those who practised what Miss Nina Morson preached in her *British Journal of Nursing* article, 'The midwife's duties to her patients', published in March 1908. They were advised to stick to a routine, to build a relationship with the mothers-to-be, and in her capacity as a health missioner, to 'try to be a power of good in every home she enters.' Midwives such as Miss Morson hardly needed inspecting, but she was the exception rather than the rule, and it was not long before inspectors were appointed countrywide to monitor standards. Many women resented the intrusion into their established working practice and private lives, which included having their homes inspected to ensure they were spotlessly clean, with well-ventilated rooms and fully functioning drains. High standards of personal hygiene were enforced to avoid infection, and midwives were advised to protect their hands getting chapped from housework, and to wear housemaid's gloves if they had to do much scrubbing, grate-cleaning or polishing. These regulations certainly had an impact but there was little that could be done to improve illiteracy among many *bona fide* midwives. This deficiency meant that many were unable to record accurate details of their cases, take a pulse, or read a thermometer. Some got around the case-note problem by making a mental note at the time and then getting a neighbour or relative to write up their notes, but the thermometer and pulse issues were potentially more serious. As *Nursing Notes* pointed out, changes in temperature and heart rate were 'the earliest and surest indication of the onset of puerperal (childbed) fever when the disease is still amenable to treatment.'

Clapham Maternity Hospital was the first of its kind, where women were treated only by female doctors and where the all-female staff were trained entirely by women.

Childbed fever was a devastating and rapidly progressive disease, which affected women within the first three days of giving birth. Many died after suffering acute symptoms of severe abdominal pain, fever and debility, but the cause remained unknown until the late 1800s, when a connection was made between germs and dirt, and a strict hygiene regime was subsequently introduced.

The fact that many midwives were unable to use a catheter may have been a blessing in disguise, for the instrument was a significant source of infection in the wrong hands. As for taking a temperature, Miss Burnside, the

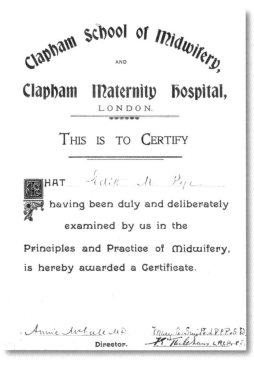

Clapham School of Midwifery,
AND
Clapham Maternity Hospital,
LONDON.

THIS IS TO CERTIFY

THAT *Edith M. Pye*
having been duly and deliberately
examined by us in the
Principles and Practice of Midwifery,
is hereby awarded a Certificate.

Annie Metcalfe M.D.
Director.

Mary ... L.R.C.P. & S.I.
... ... L.R.C.P.I.

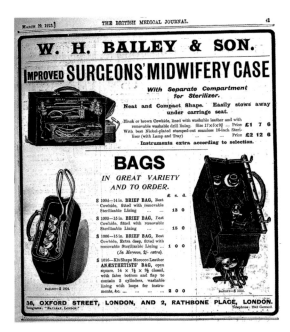

first inspector appointed in Hertfordshire, resolved the problem by getting the Medical Supply Association, a London-based supplier of medical equipment, to produce a large thermometer, clearly marked with a red line at 100.4 degrees Fahrenheit, which indicated that the doctor must be sent for. Midwifery bags became an essential item under the new rules, but they were costly, and many *bona fide* midwives continued to make do with their none-too-clean shopping baskets, carrying items such as tea, sugar and tobacco alongside some very basic equipment. They also ignored instructions to wear 'a dress of clean washable material, which can cover all,' and persisted in wearing unhygienic garments which were rarely washed and harboured germs.

The surgeon's midwifery case shown above (1913) contains forceps.

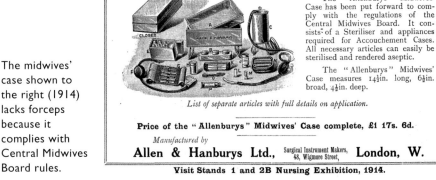

The midwives' case shown to the right (1914) lacks forceps because it complies with Central Midwives Board rules.

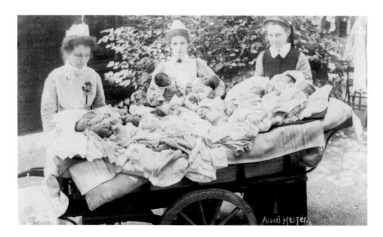

Salvation Army midwives in Hackney taking some of the babies in their care out for fresh air and sunshine, 1908.

Many midwives lived near their patients, travelling around on foot or bicycle, while those in remote areas travelled on horseback. The inspectors had a more daunting prospect, having to cover hundreds of miles across a whole county. No wonder that Miss Burnside was very relieved when, in 1913, her county council replaced her trusty bicycle with a 9.5 horse power Standard car, nicknamed 'little hero.'

A midwife sitting beside a baby in an incubator at the General Lying-in Hospital, York Road, London, 1908.

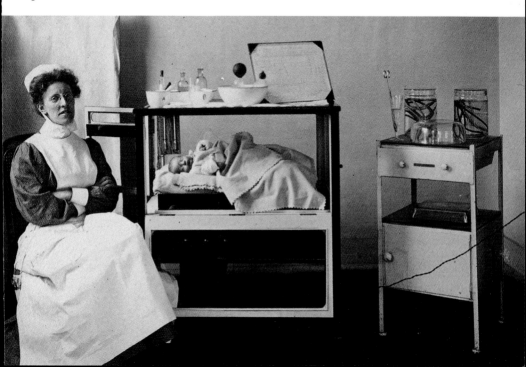

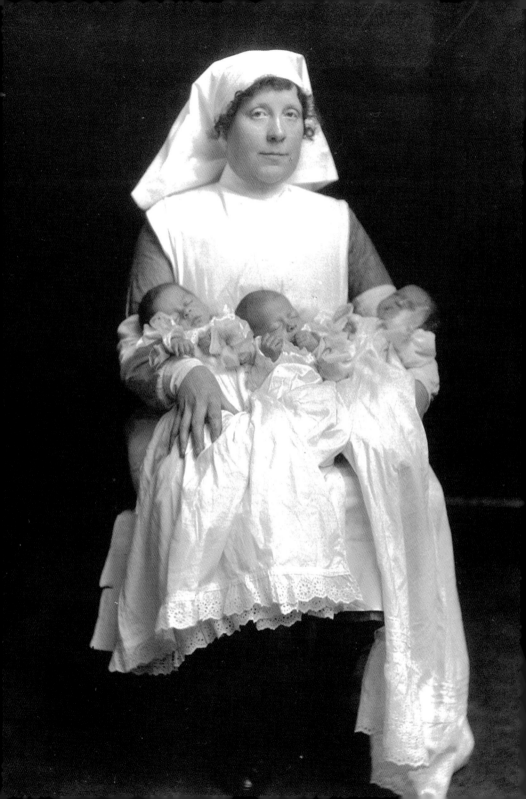

THE FIRST WORLD WAR AND BEYOND

THE ADVENT OF the First World War placed an additional burden on both midwives and expectant mothers, and many of the latter found themselves alone as their menfolk left to join the war effort. Most had home deliveries, but the wives of some absent soldiers and sailors were offered the choice of going into a lying-in (maternity) hospital for their confinement. Hospital was by no means a safer place to have a baby, but at least it enabled the mother to rest, an unlikely possibility in the homes of most, where overcrowding and ill-health were commonplace.

Many of the 386 women who wrote of their maternity experiences for the Women's Co-operative Guild in 1914 described scrimping and saving a few pence, doing heavy housework up to the moment of delivery, and having to use an untrained midwife who sometimes enlisted a child to help. Multiple births were very unusual, so much so that Queen Victoria had introduced a King's Bounty of £3 to help couples with the additional financial burden. The money was certainly welcomed by unemployed labourer William Stevenson, whose wife gave birth to triplets in Ilkeston, Derbyshire in March 1926. They were lucky that their midwife, Eveland Hutchings, applied for the grant on their behalf, and that a firm of manufacturers of a special food for babies offered a supply for as long it was needed.

Professional antenatal care was rare, and the traditional pattern in Barrow in Lancashire, replicated around the country,

Opposite: Eveland Hutchings with the Stevenson triplets, 1926. Mr Stevenson was reported as being 'obviously perplexed' by this increase in his family, stating 'When I knew it knocked me over' and that such 'family responsibilities' always seemed to befall those who could little afford it. The last of the triplets died in 2012.

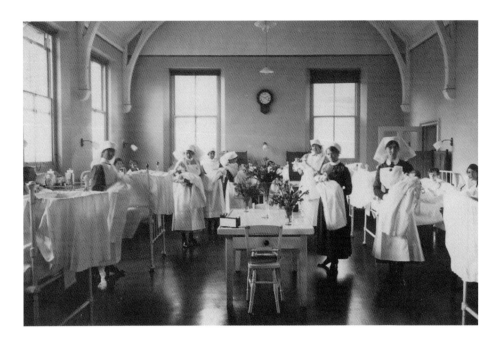

Interior of the maternity ward at Queen Charlotte's Hospital, about 1910, with some of the babies' cots hanging at the ends of the beds.

was for a woman to plan her confinement by 'booking' the midwife. In reality this meant that about the time the woman was due, the midwife would come round on a bicycle, 'and do what she had to do, you see. Examine them and say, "Oh well, when you're ready, give me a call."' For most women, childbirth was a painful experience, and midwives could do little to help them. The only concession available was chloral hydrate, a mild sedative, but as Edie B remarked, it made mothers sick almost immediately. She also recalled 'a phase where we had horrible little chloroform capsules ... you had

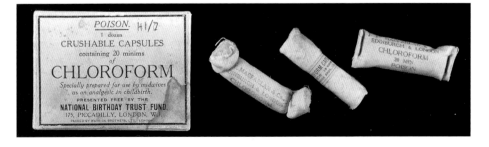

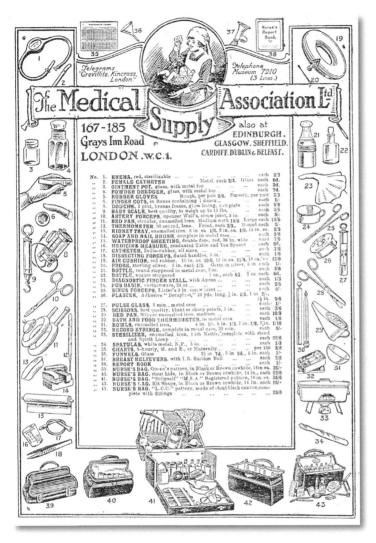

An advert in *Nursing Notes and Midwives Chronicle* showing the typical contents of a midwife's bag, November 1923.

Opposite: The use of chloroform capsules owed much to the encouragement of Miss Edith Pye, president of the Midwives' Institute from 1929.

a lint mask and you just squeezed (the content) onto the lint and put it over the mother's face every time a pain came,' but these were neither universally liked nor even safe.

It was hard for midwives to earn a living wage, and fees varied widely even within the same county. Rural midwives generally charged two or three shillings less per case than those in an urban area, but the very low rates in London

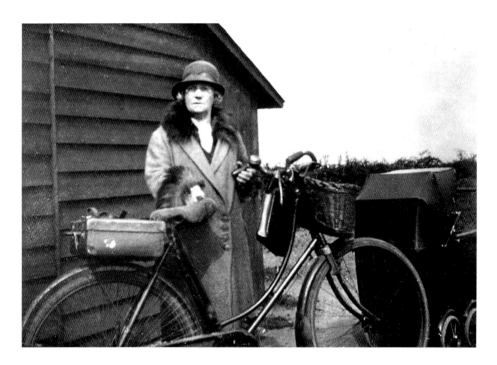

Agnes Leeden (née Green), worked as a midwife in and around the rural village of Colkirk, Norfolk, in the 1920s and 1930s.

in particular, forced midwives to take on far too many cases, putting mothers at risk. Even working for a nursing association did not guarantee financial security and one rural midwife, writing in *Nursing Notes* in the 1920s, bemoaned the fact that on her £84 a year salary she could not afford to buy a new pair of shoes, or to replace either her worn-out, leaking, rainproof coat or her three-year-old, patched, cotton work frocks. Nor did she have enough spare money to enable her 'to join the Women's Institute or anything else, and it is hard to see everybody else go off to the local entertainment and have to stay behind because of the expense.'

The economic depression of the 1930s only exacerbated matters, and the situation was especially dire in areas of high unemployment such as the Rhondda Valley in Wales. There, many local midwives could not recover any payment from the mothers, while some settled for half of what they were due. Given their poverty it is hardly surprising that many

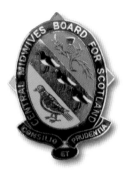
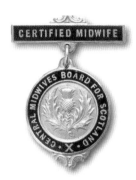
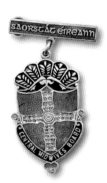

mothers chose a cheaper untrained midwife, but cost was not the only factor, for many working-class women found them to be friendlier, less 'starchy' and far less likely to tell them what to do. They also had more faith in the naturalness of their techniques, for these midwives rarely used instruments and, unlike many doctors, hardly ever inserted their hand inside a laboring woman.

Rural areas continued to suffer from a shortage of midwives and in Wiltshire in 1923, for example, only 63 per cent of outlying villages had a trained midwife, and most of the remainder had no registered midwife at all. These were lonely, isolated places to work, and presented the midwife with huge communication problems. One midwife, who had three villages in her district, was four and a half miles away from the doctor, up a very bad, uphill road. The only communication available was a single telegraph office, which was only open between 9am and 7pm. Another, Elsie B, worked in rural Scotland in the 1930s, and had to travel five miles to reach a doctor and another two miles to get to a telephone. Being called out to cases in the night meant going through woods and fields in the dark, regardless of the weather, and bikes often had to be abandoned as the roads were so muddy.

The creation of a state-salaried midwifery service after 1936 owed much to the aggressive national campaign launched by the recently established National Birthday Trust Fund

Above left: The Central Midwives Board was established in Scotland by the Midwives (Scotland) Act, 1915, and oversaw the enrolment, training and practice of midwives.

Above middle: The red enamel badge was issued to Jessie M. Bear, Roll no. 11834, on 23 July 1935.

Above right: The Central Midwives Board was established in Ireland by the Midwives Act (Ireland) of 1918.

NURSING NOTES AND MIDWIVES' CHRONICLE

A PRACTICAL JOURNAL FOR MIDWIVES AND NURSES.

BEING THE JOURNAL OF

THE INCORPORATED MIDWIVES' INSTITUTE, THE ASSOCIATION OF CERTIFIED MIDWIVES,
ITS AFFILIATED ASSOCIATIONS, AND THE TRAINED NURSES' CLUB.

THE POST CERTIFICATE SCHOOL FOR MIDWIVES.
THE ASSOCIATION FOR PROMOTING THE TRAINING AND SUPPLY OF MIDWIVES.
AND THE OVERSEAS NURSING ASSOCIATION.

Office—12, BUCKINGHAM STREET, STRAND, LONDON, W.C.2

Vol. XXXVIII.   No. 447   Entered at Stationers' Hall.   MARCH, 1925.   [Price 3d.   Post free, 4d.

CONTENTS.

MIDWIVES' INSTITUTE.

(Founded 1881. Incorporated 1880)

THE ASSOCIATION OF CERTIFIED MIDWIVES AND TRAINED NURSES' CLUB,

12, Buckingham Street, Strand, W.C.2.

March, 1925.

6th, Friday, 6.30 p.m.—Executive Council and Club Committee.

13th, Friday, 4 p.m.—Executive Council and Committee of Affiliated Associations.

20th, Friday, 6 p.m.—House Committee.

"   "   7 p.m.—Social Evening. Hostess : Miss I. Hill. Miss Marsters will speak on "Business Methods," followed by discussion.

27th, Friday, 6.30 p.m.—Midwives in Council, to discuss the results of the County Council Elections.

LECTURES to prepare for the Central Midwives Board Examination twice a week (Mondays and Wednesdays, at 5 p.m.).

MIDWIVES ASSOCIATIONS.

(Affiliated to the Midwives' Institute).

East Sussex.

The next meeting will be held on Monday, March 9th at 3.15 p.m. at the Wesleyan Schoolroom, Perrymount Road, Hayward's Heath, when Miss Cancellor of the N.C.C.V.D. will speak on Venereal Disease as a Complication of & Pregnancy.—E. M. Wyatt, Hon. Sec.

Birmingham.

March 13th, Dr. Dain, 4.45 p.m. Subject : Menopause and Cancer. —Miss Rickford, Secretary.

Blackpool and District.

The next meeting will be Wednesday, March 11th, 3 p.m.—M. Lightbown, Hon. Sec.

Bournemouth.

A meeting will be held at the G.F.S. Club, St. Peter's Road on Monday, March 2nd, at 3 p.m. Tea 6d. Speaker Miss Maude Hone, M.B., Ch.B.—I. M. C. Druitt, Hon. Sec.

Bristol.

The next meeting will be held at the Kingswood Nurses Home, Hanham Road, by kind invitation of Miss Bosworth, on March 17th, at 3.30 p.m. An address will be given by Miss Cross (Matron of The Maternity Hospital, Brunswick Square). "A Short Talk about Midwifery in Italy."—Miss Hancock, Hon. Sec.

Gosport and Fareham.

The meeting for March will be held at the "House of Industry," Gosport, 3 p.m., on the 18th. Dr. Una Mulvany of Portsmouth will Lecture. Any midwife visiting the district will be welcome.— L. M. Cryer, Hon. Sec.

ESSEX.

Southend Branch.

Wednesday, March 18th, Dr. C. A. Shields, Public Health Office, Clarence Street, 3.15 p.m.—Mrs. Tween, Secretary, 85, Stornaway Road, Southchurch.

Colchester Branch.

Tuesday, March 17th, Dr. Ryan. Ear, Nose and Throat, 71, High Street, Colchester, 3 p.m.—Miss Pearson, Secretary, Health Offices, Colchester.

Chelmsford Branch.

Saturday, March 7th, Miss Burdew, Nursing of "Chronics," 3 p.m., 125 London Road.—Nurse N. Millett, Secretary.

S.E. Essex Branch.

Friday, March 13th, Miss Elsie Hall, the Midwives Opportunity. Nurses' Home, Beachcroft Road, Leytonstone, 5.30 p.m.—Nurse Kennard, Secretary.

Saffron Waldon Branch.

Tuesday, March 17th, Miss Landon, Antenatal Work, 37, West Road, 3 p.m.—Nurse Doyle and Nurse Crampton, Secretaries.

Romford Branch.

Wednesday, March 11th, Dr. Ball, Infant Feeding, Tuberculosis Dispensary, 3 p.m.—Miss Landon, Secretary, Old Cottage, Shenfield Common, Brentwood.

Hertfordshire.

A course of lectures is being given monthly by Dr. Helen Noth, at Bricket House, St. Albans, at 3.30 p.m. Next one March 19th. Tea provided after each lecture.—E. S. Cowper, Hon. Sec.

Liverpool.

March 12th : "Disorders of the Climacteric," Miss Ivens, University of Liverpool, Department of Hygiene. March 26th : "Prevention of Ophthalmia Neonatorum," Dr. T. Stevenson, St. Paul's Eye Hospital.

Maidstone.

Tuesday, March 3rd, at 3 p.m., at Sessions House, Dr. Ponder, Assist. M.O.H., will lecture on the Infant.—H. Wells, Hon. Sec.

Portsmouth.

Next meeting at Welfare Centre, Fratton Road on Wednesday, March 4th, 3.45 p.m. Lecture by Dr. McCalden, Subject : "Twilight Sleep."—A. G. Phillips, Hon. Sec.

Whitefield and District.

March 12th, a lecture will be given by Dr. Hall at 2.45 p.m.—A. J. P. Hon. Sec.

S.W. London.

A Social will be held on Monday, March 2nd, at 7 p.m., at 47 Lavender Gardens. Members and friends are invited.—C. A. Tiffin, Hon. Sec.

Southampton and District.

A meeting will be held at the Municipal Clinic on Wednesday, March 11th, at 6 p.m. Report of Representative.—E. Harvey, Hon. Sec.

Cornwall.

The next meeting will be on Saturday, March 28th, at the Infant Welfare Centre, Lemon Quay, Truro, at 3. p.m. Lecture by Dr. Burnell commencing 3.15 p.m.—Ethel Lyon, Hon. Sec.

North Middlesex.

Next meeting Wednesday, March 11th, at 260, Fore Street, Edmonton. Dr. Ash will give his second lecture, which unavoidably had to be postponed.—M. Andrews, Hon. Sec.

for Maternity Services. Their intervention led to the Midwives Act being revised in 1936, and with the exception of women who chose to remain independent, midwives now had the advantage, in theory, of a secure salary, guaranteed three weeks' annual leave and inclusion in a pension scheme. However, they were still responsible for collecting their fee, which proved difficult when so many clients were poor. On the plus side, they were now provided with a uniform, equipment, a laundry allowance and a bicycle, and there was also the promise of a half-day off a week, although this did not always materialise. As Mary W recalled, 'If you'd a lot of deliveries – a lot of nights up, no one made it up for you, you just had to go on and get it over and get your sleep when you could. I remember one week when I didn't see my husband to speak to.'

The new act also benefited mothers, for it enabled midwives with the appropriate qualifications to administer inhalation anaesthesia. The Minnitt gas and air (nitrous-oxide/oxygen) machine eventually transformed pain relief, but there were midwives who were reluctant to use it, believing, like Elizabeth C, that the best form of pain

*The
Expectant
Mother*

Published by the
NATIONAL BIRTHDAY TRUST FUND
(for Extension of Maternity Services)
57, LOWER BELGRAVE STREET,
LONDON, S.W.1

Artwork for the cover of a series of lectures given by the National Birthday Trust Fund, and donation cards.

Opposite: Front cover of the Midwives' Institute monthly journal (March 1925).

CENTRAL MIDWIVES BOARD

This is to certify that the

City of London Maternity Hospital

has notified the Central Midwives Board that

Grace Cécile Moore

No. *109666*

has completed the prescribed training at the institution in the administration of nitrous oxide and air by means of *Minnitt's Apparatus* (an apparatus recognized by the Central Midwives Board as suitable for use by midwives, under the conditions prescribed by the Board, for the purpose of producing analgesia during childbirth). In connexion therewith she has received special instruction in the essentials of obstetric analgesia and in the emergencies of anæsthesia, adequate for such purpose, and has been found, after examination, to be thoroughly proficient in the use of the apparatus under the conditions prescribed by the Central Midwives Board.

P. Bennett
Secretary.

Date *30th June 1946*

Midwives had to attend the officially prescribed number of cases before they were awarded their certificate allowing them to administer anaesthesia.

relief came from 'knowing the midwife, it's better than dope or something because it's a normal thing, you see.' Her views echoed those of Dr Grantly Dick-Read (1890–1959) whose first book, *Natural Childbirth*, was published in 1933, and which in turn, influenced the founders of the National Childbirth Association, subsequently Trust, in 1956.

What midwives did not have was access to any oxygen or resuscitation equipment, so they had a variety of ways of 'persuading' a reluctant newborn baby to take a first breath. The popular method was to hold a baby by its feet, but Margaret A offered the alternatives of 'taking hold of the feet and pat the bottom of its feet – or another thing, too – blow in the centre of their tummies.' What she would not do was emulate a doctor whom she had seen blow cigarette smoke in the baby's face, on the grounds that it probably irritated the mucous membranes.

War was looming, and during 1938 and early 1939 an increasing number of young Jewish women refugees arrived in Britain from Germany, Austria and Czechoslovakia, seeking a safe haven from Nazi persecution. Miss Edith Pye, the president of the Midwives' Institute, was proactive in enabling some who were partially trained to complete their midwifery training in Britain and gain employment.

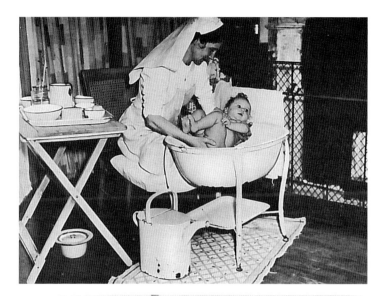

An illustration from Mabel Liddiard's bestselling book, *The Mothercraft Manual*, first published in 1923. Here the midwife is demonstrating how to lift a baby into a bath.

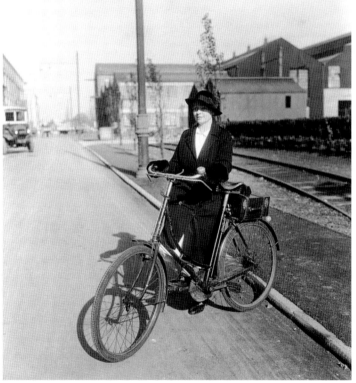

A midwife transporting an analgesic gas and air machine by bicycle, about 1937. The early machines, prior to this one, were costly, bulky and too heavy for most midwives to transport by bicycle or on foot.

A NEW TRAINING REGIME

DESPITE THE NATIONWIDE shortage of midwives, keen working-class women continued to find it difficult to qualify throughout the 1920s and 1930s. Funding was a huge factor, for they had to find money for their uniform, equipment, exam and tuition fees. Mary W, a trained nurse, found a solution to the latter by working unpaid at a nursing home for six months, in lieu of tuition fees, before embarking on her course in 1931. Some women resorted to training at fever and tuberculosis hospitals where any willing applicant was welcomed, providing they were prepared to risk their health while gaining some nursing experience. Training courses began to develop in 1926, with pupil midwives spending a maximum of one year in training, depending on their background. Theory was taught in thirty lectures, and practice required them to supervise and care for twenty women, before, during and after childbirth. The course itself could be a daunting experience, with pupil midwives subjected to the authority of their tutor. Mary Thomson found her initiation at Rotten Row hospital, Glasgow, in the early 1930s humiliating and exhausting, and shattered her illusions of becoming 'a ministering angel on a mission of mercy.'

CMB certificate, 1926.

No. *18950*   Date *April 29th 19 26*

Central Midwives Board.
[2 Edw. VII. Ch. 17]

We hereby Certify

That   *Annie Harding*

having passed the Examination of the Central Midwives Board, and having otherwise complied with the rules and regulations laid down in pursuance of the Midwives Act, 1902, is entitled by law to practise as a Midwife in accordance with the provisions of the said Act and subject to the said rules and regulations.

F.H. Champneys
Chairman of the Board.

Secretary.

Florence was another who recalled feeling inferior because of her lack of formal education, remarking 'although you had the experience those nurses hadn't in life and that, you didn't have the head knowledge.' When it came to taking the CMB exam, quite a number of girls travelled north to Scotland where the fees at 'Old Simpson', officially the Edinburgh Royal Maternity and Simpson Memorial Hospital, were set at £45 in 1935, considerably lower than the £62 being charged at Queen Charlotte's in London.

The biggest change came in 1938 when the course was extended and divided into two, with an exam taken after the completion of each part. The new part one combined theoretical and practical training, and took place in the maternity hospital setting, with shifts spent in antenatal, labour and postnatal wards. Subjects covered in the compulsory forty lectures included elementary anatomy and physiology, as well as hygiene and sanitation and their relationship to normal pregnancy, childbirth and the care of infants. Great emphasis was put on the midwife's place in the medical hierarchy, and although pupils could be taught about a specific obstetric operation, it was made clear that they would only ever be called upon to act as a skilled assistant to a doctor. There were strict rules of etiquette to follow, and when a doctor came onto the ward, the students would all stand to attention. Similarly they were expected to open and close ward doors for

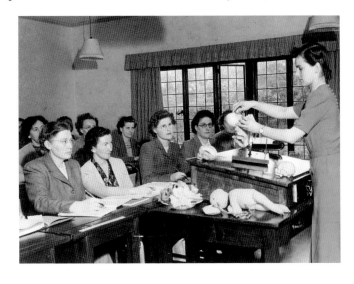

A student, Betty Lowe, giving a practice teaching class, 1 September 1950.

REGISTER OF CASES.

Entries in Grace Moore's case book as a pupil midwife at the East End Maternity Hospital, London in 1941. Grace, was also a district nurse, additionally trained by the Queen Victoria Jubilee Institute for Nurses, and during the Second World War became known as the 'Midwife of Petticoat Lane'.

him, keep the patients quiet during rounds and make sure he had clean hot water.

Much of the training was routine, from making beds to cleaning instruments, and Mrs S recalled how, in the days before pre-packed equipment, syringes had to be washed and put in spirit, ready for use. Keeping the mother clean was vital and to this end a gowned and masked pupil was shown how to sit the mother on a sterile bed pan, and after ablutions were completed, to 'wash them (the mother) from the umbilicus to the knee with, we called them bottom bowls … then either you or someone else came round with the swabbing trolley and they were swabbed down.' Miss P was not the only trainee to comment that the worst day for bedpan duty was on the second night after delivery, when a mother was given half a cup of liquorice powder to make sure her bowels worked.

Living in close quarters with their fellow students during training helped develop a sense of professional identity, duty and responsibility, and many women thoroughly enjoyed the camaraderie. One recorded how 'there was quite a lot of fun really and we shared everybody else's romance or whatever was going on.' While Matron would not eat in the same dining room as the other staff, the students liked the attention they got from the maids, especially on their days off, when breakfast might be delivered to their bedroom. Part two of training was six months spent delivering babies, either totally 'on the district' or divided between home deliveries and a maternity ward. This was particularly hard work. Along with many other requirements, including five lectures and sessions at an infant and maternal welfare clinic, the rules stipulated responsibility for a minimum of twenty labours, half of which had to be in the home. However, the demands were so great that some pupils attended as many as ten a month, with one pupil recalling that 'you could go from one delivery to another in the night and maybe end up with two or three deliveries.'

From going out with a midwife to taking sole care of a mother and her delivery was a big step forward, and students were only meant to call the tutor out if they needed a second opinion. Having sole charge for several women all due to

Midwives getting ready to leave the nurses' home, c. 1950s.

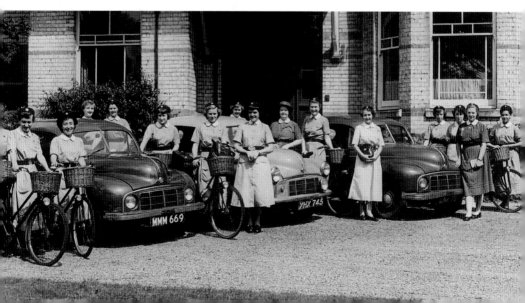

The Organisers of the

Twenty-Fifth Nursing and Midwifery Exhibition

New Horticultural Hall, Westminster.

(Nearest Station : St. James's Park)

March 11, 12, 13, 14 and 15th, 1935
11 a.m. to 7 p.m. daily

First Day opening 2.30.   Last Day closing 6 p.m.

Extend a hearty invitation to all Midwives to visit the Exhibition, which will be wholly re-organised.

Applicants for tickets should enclose 3d. in stamps for registration and postage, and should state their PERMANENT Address. The tickets when presented at the Exhibition, and officially stamped will admit to all Sessions of the Conference.

REFRESHMENTS   ORCHESTRA

SISTER TUTOR'S LECTURE ROOM

Apply The Ticket Bureau,
NURSING and MIDWIFERY EXHIBITION,
40, HOLLAND PARK, W. 11.
Telephone : PARK 6073

deliver around the same time could be very taxing, and a midwife might be up for two or three consecutive nights. One pupil was so tired she recalled going to sleep momentarily on her bike. Mary Cronk, a pupil midwife in Paisley, near Glasgow in 1955, recalled carrying around a 'very rough and ready' portable kit which included 'urine- and blood-testing equipment' and, in the days before ultrasound scans and the like, a fetal stethoscope. 'We were taught how to listen to the baby's heartbeat. I also carried shillings for the electricity meter and pennies for the phone box.' Without scales to hand, she would weigh a newborn baby in a nappy using a spring weighing device.

'On the district' students typically lived in the nurses' home, which varied in quality. One in Hull left a lasting memory with the pupils, for it was flea-ridden, which the students blamed on their poverty-stricken patients whose homes were often infested, and far from hygienic. Mary Cronk was quickly made all too aware of the deprivation in Glasgow when she made an antenatal visit to see if the surroundings were suitable for a home delivery. 'A bathroom with hot and cold running water was a luxury. They would drink out of jam jars or cups without handles but would always manage to borrow a cup and saucer for the midwife.' Superstitions still prevailed as Mary soon discovered: 'Quite often a young neighbour would appear asking if she could stay because there was a legend that if the afterbirth popped and crackled, someone else in the room would have a baby within a year.'

Any notion that the pupil midwife's day was finished after her rounds were complete was an illusion, for there was a mountain of work to do to prepare for the night and day ahead. Bags had to be stripped down, enamel bowls and gloves boiled, aprons washed, and the bag repacked. Then there were the records of the women attended to be brought up to date; these were subject to regular inspection by the supervisor who would order untidy ones to be rewritten. Tired pupils dreaded the night-time phone calls, one even revealing how she tried to persuade mothers that they were not really in labour. She would say 'Are you sure you've started? Are they regular? Oh, they aren't very strong yet are they?' – putting off getting out of bed as long as possible.

The newly qualified midwife used all the knowledge acquired during her training, and refined it further as she became more experienced. No self-respecting midwife would allow a mother to tear the perineum, which would then need the doctor to attend to apply sutures. The sign of a well-managed labour and of good practice was one where the midwife encouraged slow, steady deliveries, allowing natural stretching. Sissy S, whose babies were born in the 1920s and 1930s, recalled always being told 'to lie on your left side and "Steady, steady … that's right – now bear down, slowly … slowly … now the next pain is going to be very hard…" …I never tore with any of my babies. Not even the one that was 12 pounds.' She never needed a doctor, but midwives understood the boundaries of their role and as one commented, 'the art is knowing when things are going wrong.' By the end of the 1930s, it was not only pupils who had to undergo training, for the first of the new residential refresher courses for practising midwives was planned for September 1939, but were postponed because of the outbreak of war.

Opposite: An advertisement in *Nursing Notes* for the twenty-fifth Nursing and Midwifery Exhibition in March 1935. The annual exhibition was a big event in the nursing calendar, but was suspended during the war years.

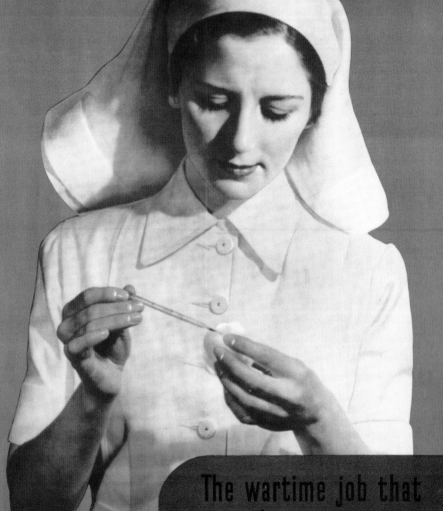

NURSES & Midwives are needed

The wartime job that can be your career

ENQUIRE AT THE NEAREST APPOINTMENTS OFFICE OF THE MINISTRY OF LABOUR & NATIONAL SERVICE OR WRITE TO: 24 KINGSWAY, LONDON, W.C.2

PRINTED FOR H.M. STATIONERY OFFICE BY J. WEINER LTD, LONDON. WC1 51-1642

THE SECOND WORLD WAR

WHILE THE COUNTRY braced itself for bombing and invasion, the Midwives' Institute campaigned for steel helmets and respirators for their members, and many midwives in rural areas found themselves acting as surrogate mothers to children evacuated from the cities. The profession was designated high priority by the government during the war years, but the inherent shortage of midwives was compounded as many medical staff were called up for military service. Added to this, some nurse-trained midwives were tempted to join as reservists with, amongst other organisations, Queen Alexandra's Imperial Military Nursing Service (QAIMNS), either because they wanted to help the war effort or because, as Jean Woods recalled, they found the prospect of official recognition and a decorated uniform 'enticing'. Pat Lawrence was turned down by the QAIMNS because of her poor eyesight, and instead undertook a six-month midwifery course in Bristol so she could join the colonial service after the war. She recalled, 'We had lectures at the hospital and went out to antenatal clinics in different parts of the city where we examined the expectant mothers under the watchful eye of the doctor in charge and an experienced midwife.'

Long hours and hardship became commonplace as midwives struggled to cope with an unprecedented increase in the birth rate, which peaked in 1946. As one midwife whom Lindsay Reid interviewed remarked, 'The birth rate always went up after the men had been home on leave.'

Opposite:
A wartime poster for the government's campaign to retain nurses and midwives on the home front.

Midwife and assistants in the Lincolnshire fens, 1939. The midwife would deliver the baby then give it to one of the girls to clear the nose and eyes, and give it a slap on the back to make sure it was breathing.

To ease the crisis, independent midwives were urged to enrol with the CMB if they were willing to offer their services in an emergency. Those whose skills were a bit rusty could take advantage of the short refresher courses which became available around the country, courtesy of the Midwives' Institute, which became the College of Midwives in 1941. Then, in 1943, the government issued an order which required anyone who was or had been a nurse or midwife to register at an employment exchange, effectively preventing them enlisting. However, as Jean Woods also recalled, some pupil midwives in Glasgow got around this by interrupting their training after completing part one of the syllabus to enlist. The employment exchanges also took over responsibility for placing midwives around the country, with the aim of overcoming geographical shortages. But a proposal that first-aiders should be given instruction on attending confinements was dismissed out of hand by the Midwives' Institute as both dangerous and unnecessary.

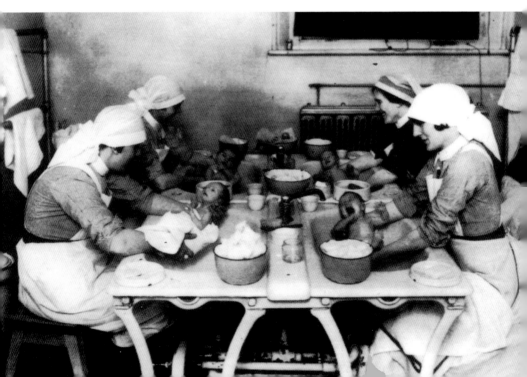

For those caught up in the Blitz, danger was never far away, and the start of an air raid was sometimes enough to precipitate a woman's labour. It also prevented a mother being moved to the safety of an air-raid shelter, in which case any protection would do. The renamed *Midwives Chronicle and Nursing Notes* reported in September 1941 of a London baby born in a cupboard, 'to the accompaniment of gunfire and several heavy explosions, falling plaster and rocking house.' As the baby was about to be delivered, a pilotless bomb fell nearby, and the quick-thinking midwife covered the mother's face with a pillow and the oncoming infant with her tin hat, protecting them both from glass and plaster. Bristol was equally unsafe, and the journal recorded how midwives Mrs E. Rice and Miss Victoria Frampton dodged bombs and flying masonry to find a pregnant woman trapped underneath debris. They stayed with her for hours while a rescue team worked to release her; she was then transferred to hospital and her baby safely delivered. Mrs Rice was awarded the George Medal in March 1941 for her bravery. Helen Owen, a Red Cross volunteer who assisted midwife Sister Middleton in the remote Lincolnshire fens, faced a different kind of hazard, for the Austin 7 the women travelled in often ended up in a ditch, and had to be hauled out by a farm tractor.

Many inner-city maternity homes were relocated to the relative safety of the countryside but the urban mothers disliked being forced to live in the country. Carloads of expectant mothers were sent from London to one of Lord Rothschild's homes near Tring every week, but as midwife Edie B recalled they used to say 'We cannot stand this 'orrible 'ush. Somebody rattle a tin can or something!' According to midwife Florence W, what they really missed were 'bingo, fish and chips and the cinema.' The midwives themselves held varying opinions and while Esther S loved being in the country, especially enjoying the walks, Nellie H found

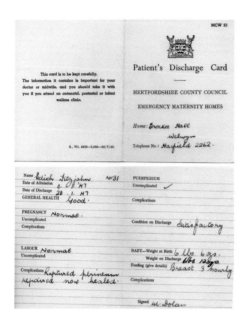

Patient's Discharge Card

HERTFORDSHIRE COUNTY COUNCIL

EMERGENCY MATERNITY HOMES

Home: Brocket Hall Welwyn

Telephone No.: Hatfield 2262.

This card is to be kept carefully. The information it contains is important for your doctor or midwife, and you should take it with you if you attend an antenatal, postnatal or infant welfare clinic.

S., Wt. 2629—2,000—25/7/45.

MCW 23

Name Edith Fitzjohn   Apr 31

Date of Admission 11-01-47

Date of Discharge 28.1.47

GENERAL HEALTH Good.

PREGNANCY Normal.
Uncomplicated
Complications

LABOUR Normal
Uncomplicated

Complications Ruptured perineum repaired now healed.

PUERPERIUM
Uncomplicated ✓

Complications

Condition on Discharge Satisfactory

BABY—Weight at Birth 6 lbs. 6 ozs.
Weight on Discharge 6 lbs 12 ozs
Feeding (give details) Breast 3 hourly

Complications

Signed M. Dolan

Brocket Hall, Hertfordshire, became home to the London Maternity Hospital between 1939 and 1949. Evacuated mothers spent up to ten days recovering from childbirth in luxurious surroundings.

the experience very disruptive, even though she loved the wartime spirit and camaraderie. One hospital that continued to function in London was the Hackney-based Salvation Army Mothers' Hospital. With speedy evacuation in mind, the midwives got the mothers out of bed within two days of delivery, so that they could get to the specially constructed underground shelters in the grounds more quickly. An indirect benefit of early ambulation was a decrease in cases of postnatal deep vein thrombosis, generally brought about by inactivity, and was a practice that many midwives, including Margaret A, continued after the war, well before it became general policy.

The hard-pressed midwives dealt with labour and deliveries, a considerable amount of domestic work, as well as staffing the nursery. Pupil midwife Pat Lawrence recalled that, in the hospital in Bristol where she worked in 1944, the babies were fed every three hours. Breastfeeding was the norm, and bottles were only ever suggested for the baby of a very sick mother, or one with a serious underlying medical condition.

Midwives gradually had a range of new drugs available to counteract infection and control bleeding, as well as the introduction of a blood transfusion service. They also had access to obstetric 'flying squads', which came out from the hospital with staff and equipment to help them deal with a home emergency. These developed in the 1930s, with Bellshill, Lanarkshire operating a service in 1931. The Newcastle-upon-Tyne service dealt with one case in 1935 and with forty-six by 1938, becoming the role model for others.

LABOUR WARD NOTES.

Name and Age	... ...	*Mrs Edith Pearce 26.* Husband's Name. *occupation*
Address	... ...	*146. West Raw Drive. William Jones. Engineer.* *Barking.*
Religion	... ...	*Methodist*

		MEASUREMENTS.	
Date of Admission	... *23. 5. 41.*	**PELVIS :—**	**UTERUS :—**
Number of Prev. Pregs.	... *0.*	External Conjugate *8"*	Height
PAINS Began	... *2-7-41. 4.41. 4.30 p.m.*	Interspinous *9½"*	Circumference
Presentation	... *Vertex LOP-LOA*	Intercristal *11"*	
2nd Stage	... *4. 4. 41. 11.20 p.m*	Diagonal Conjugate	
Rupture of Membranes	... *4. 4. 41. 11.20 am*	True Conjugate	
Delivery of Child	.. *8. 4. 41. 12.25 am.*	**CHILD :—**	**HEAD :—**
Delivery of Placenta	... *8. 4. 41. 12. 20 am.*		Circumference
	1st. 2nd. 3rd.		B P *4½*
Labour	... ...	Sex *Female.*	B T *3½*
	3h. 50m. 45 mins 15 mins	Length *20.*	O M *5.¼*
		Weight *4. 5½*	O F *4¾*
		Receiver *4½*	S O F *4½*
Rupture of Perinæum	*2nd degree.*	*6.14*	

Date and Time	... *8-7-41. 3.30am.*							
PULSE	... ... *80*							
TEMPERATURE	... *100*							
TONGUE	... ... *clean*							
BOWELS	... *BNO*							
URINE	... *N3 Uni*							

REMARKS :— *on inspection. Smooth oval tumour.*
Palpation. 3 fingers admitted below easily on each side.
Lie longitudinal, vertex presenting. Head engaged.
Foetal back to the left & posterior. limbs to right.
Auscultation. Foetal heart heard in left flank.
Vulval exam.   Examined by :—

Labour ward notes. Notes like these were routinely kept to record all aspects of each hospital birth.

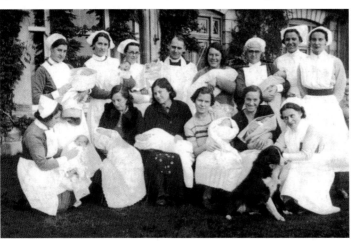

Mothers, babies and staff with the Rector W. E. Pilling, outside Whatton House, Leicestershire, November 1940. Lord and Lady Crawshaw's stately home became a maternity hospital to mothers from London and Birmingham between October 1940 and March 1945.

POST-WAR AND THE
NATIONAL HEALTH SERVICE

ABOUT SIXTY MIDWIVES joined the Victory Parade in London on 8 June 1946, and although midwifery was the most popular of the special fields of nursing service, there was still a severe shortage of practitioners. Despite their matchless skills and knowledge and the immeasurable responsibility they had of delivering babies, their profile remained low. The advent of a national uniform did help to create an identity, and in November 1946, the campaign spearheaded by the College of Midwives reached a successful conclusion, with the unveiling, at the Professional Nurses and Midwives Annual Exhibition at Seymour Hall, London, of outfits for every occasion. Mona Williams, who became a pupil midwife in a poor area of Manchester in October 1948, treasured hers, especially the dark grey woollen winter coat with its blue collar trim and SCM (State Certified Midwife) embossed buttons, and she still had it in 2011, more than thirty years after she had retired. At work, light-blue cotton dresses with a starched apron were covered with a separate clean gown to prevent cross-infection, precipitating a lot of washing, and Mona was grateful that her mother did all her laundry for her. Several midwives who were handy with a needle and thread asked for paper patterns to be made available but were told that this would 'lead to variations from the approved style.'

The establishment of the National Health Service (NHS) on 5 July 1948 heralded free medical care for all, and, in theory, any expectant mother could summon a doctor, free of charge,

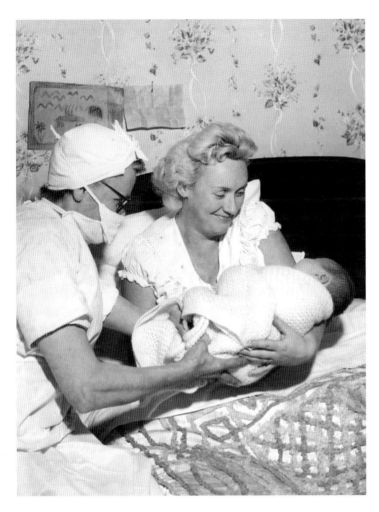

In the 1950s, this newly delivered mother would have been confined to bed for ten days, and the midwife would be involved in bed-making, bathing the baby and swabbing the mother for eight days. But for many hard-working mothers, this period of rest was all they were ever likely to get, and for that reason alone it was strictly enforced by midwives.

to attend them in childbirth. This prompted fears, articulated by the president of the Royal College of Obstetricians and Gynaecologists in *The Times* on 7 July 1948, that the role of the midwife would be taken over by medical practitioners, and their status reduced to that of a maternity nurse. Because of the pressure on doctors, these fears proved to be groundless, and although most women asked for a doctor and a midwife to attend them, in 75 per cent of cases it was the midwife who assisted them. So, even though maternal care within the new

For midwives who had not attended the exhibition, this article in *Nursing Notes* in November 1946 was the first glimpse they got of their new national uniform.

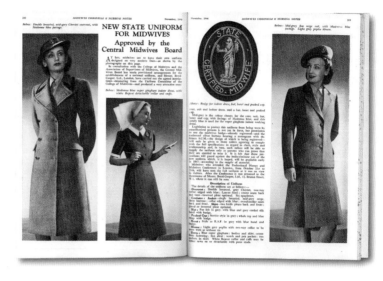

NHS was to be shared between GPs, hospital services and local authority health services, the division between hospital and district work remained.

Improvements in pay were clearly welcomed by Mona Williams. She recalled that as a nurse working before the

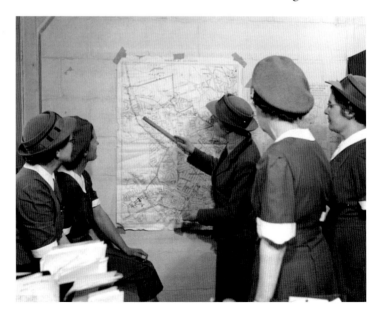

Some community midwives discussing the problems in an inner-city area before going on their rounds, about 1952.

Second World War she had been earning £20 a year, but under the NHS she received £8 a month during her midwifery training, a sum which increased to £24 a month when she qualified. There were, as she pointed out, some unwanted consequences of the new free service for she found some mothers 'were a bit demanding at first', even calling for an ambulance to take them to a hospital-booked delivery when they certainly did not need it. By the time she retired in 1978, Mona had delivered more than seven thousand babies.

Community midwives preparing their midwifery bags before leaving to make house calls in the 1950s.

The new NHS started to run campaigns to persuade mothers to have hospital confinements, but given the shortage of beds, mothers who were considered low-risk were still able

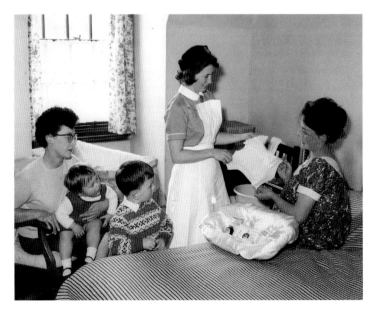

An antenatal visit by a midwife of the Queen's Nursing Institute, 1950s.

to have their babies at home. Many of them were among the most deprived in society, and lived in homes that were quite unfit for a confinement, presenting midwives with a real challenge. There were times when Dot May Dunn, working in a Midlands slum in the mid-1950s, had to use her emergency money to replenish the gas meter. If she needed a doctor in an emergency, she had to find someone to act as a messenger as there was no telephone nearby. On one occasion she resorted to calling out the 'flying squad', and was relieved when her decision was later vindicated by the general practitioner. Like most midwives, Dot got around her district by bicycle, but in the Midlands in 1951 she could not safely leave hers outside a

This community midwife was using one of the early model scooters to get around her district, c. 1950s.

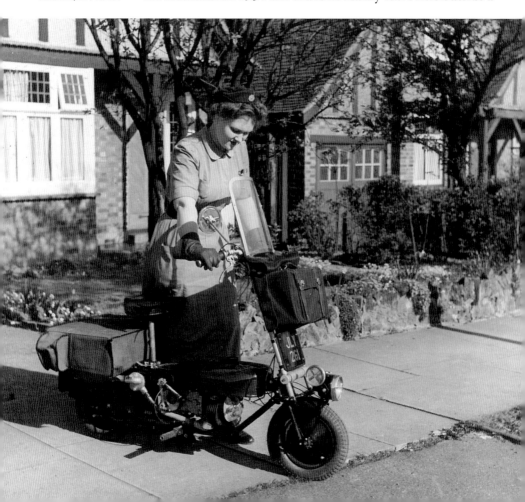

property. Instead she had to manoeuvre it, equipment and all, up and down the stairs of a lodging house so she could take it inside the mother's flat.

The dreadful winter of 1947 was the last straw for two midwives in East Anglia, and they were prepared to leave their jobs rather than face the prospect of cycling around their district again the following year in snow and ice. For them, the provision of a car to transport them and all their equipment was a dream come true, but there were other midwives, like Mary W, who missed the familiar banter directed at them as they cycled around their district.

The Community of St John the Divine where Jennifer Worth (then Lee) was initially a lay pupil midwife covered the eight-mile-square district of Poplar, one of the poorest areas in post-war London. Between eighty and a hundred babies were born there every month in the most poverty-stricken conditions. Families were crammed into tiny

Below left: The London Underground was a useful form of transport for this midwife, working in Manor House, north London, about 1950.

Below: A district midwife hands over a premature baby to the emergency paediatric service, c. 1960s.

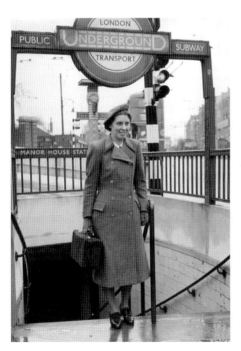

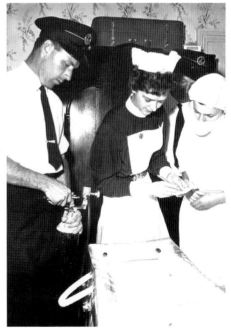

tenement houses, most of which lacked bathrooms, indoor toilets and running hot water. As viewers saw in *Call the Midwife*, the popular TV dramatisation of Jennifer Worth's memoirs, the young Poplar midwives had to learn the art of improvisation. The top of a chest of drawers would be utilised as a work surface and large sheets of non-absorbent brown paper, which she thought 'absurdly old-fashioned', served as an effective protective layer over the bed. This had the added advantage of being disposable later on, by burning, along with all the other waste items.

Mary White did her 'on the district' training in Norwich in 1947, and used a sterilised biscuit tin for keeping pads and dressings in. In homes lacking any crockery, midwives such as Mary White, Jennifer Worth and others were quite happy to accept a cup of tea served in a jam jar or even an old tin can.

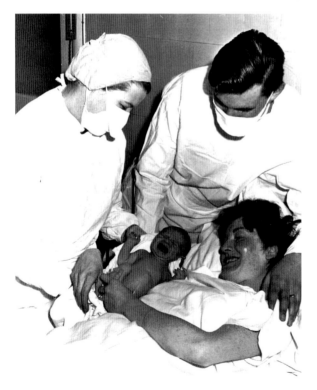

A father present at the hospital birth of his baby in the 1960s.

While rationing was still in effect, midwives had to sign 'sheet dockets' to enable a mother to get three sheets for herself and the baby, and although these were only supposed to be given in needy cases, the midwives in Sheffield disregarded this injunction, and issued them wholesale, considering every mother to be a needy case. With coal still rationed until mid-1958, Mona Wilson was not the only midwife to carry special certificates with her to ensure that new mothers had enough fuel to heat their homes. Mary Cronk began practising as a domiciliary midwife in 1959 and recalled, from her case register, that blood was routinely given on her district, East Twickenham, when mothers had a postpartum haemorrhage. The nearest blood bank was at the West Middlesex Hospital, and she would 'summon the GP who would get the blood out by ambulance', or if Mary thought it an emergency, she would 'get the blood out by ambulance to meet the GP.' She also routinely gave mothers pethidine for pain relief.

This midwife's case notes include her pre-delivery assessment of home conditions, January 1947.

HOME CONDITIONS
(TO BE COMPLETED IN THE CASE OF A DISTRICT CONFINEMENT ONLY)

SITUATION OF THE DWELLING (Basement, ground floor, first floor, etc.): Council house. One floor.

PREPARATIONS FOR THE MOTHER: Everything ready. Clean linen and clothes. Maternity box

GENERAL CONDITION (Clean, damp, in need of repair, nature of sanitation, etc.): Clean and dry. In good repair. Flush lavatory and bathroom on ground floor.

PREPARATIONS FOR THE CHILD: Basket cot warm and comfortable. Clothing and toilet requisites ready.

NAME AND ADDRESS OF " HOME HELP "

WATER SUPPLY: Main   **RENT:** 12/6.

PATIENT'S BEDROOM: Front room on 1st floor. Double bed. Electric light. Coal fire.

NUMBER OF OTHER OCCUPANTS IN ROOM 1   **NUMBER IN FAMILY** 4.

NAME OF THE DOCTOR, IF SUMMONED

SOCIAL SERVICES REQUIRED: Fuel forms. Steel tablets. Orange juice. Cod liver oil. Extra milk and eggs.

CONFINEMENT IN INSTITUTION or **IN PATIENT'S HOME:** Patient's home.

LABOUR	BEGAN	MEMBRANES RUPTURED	CERVIX FULLY DILATED	CHILD BORN	PLACENTA EXPELLED	DURATION OF LABOUR
DATE	10·1·47.	10·1·47	10·1·47	11·1·47	11·1·47	1ST STAGE 9h. 50 minutes
						2ND STAGE 25 minutes
HOUR	2 pm	12 m.n.	11.50 pm	12.15 a.m.	12.40 a.m.	3RD STAGE 35 minutes
						TOTAL 10h 60 minutes

POSITION OF CHILD: L.O.A.   **PRESENTATION:** Vertex.

PLACENTA AND MEMBRANES: METHOD OF EXPULSION: By fundal pressure from very separation.

LACERATIONS: 1ST   2ND   3RD DEGREE   **INTACT OR IMPERFECT:** Intact

RUPTURE OF PERINEUM

NUMBER OF SUTURES   **HAEMORRHAGE:** ʒ XII

	FIRST STAGE							SECOND STAGE		
DATE	10·1·47	10·1·47	10·1·47	10·1·47	10·1·47			10·1·47	10·1·47	
TIME	2 pm	3·4 pm	6 pm	8 pm	11 pm			11.50 pm	12 m.n.	
TEMPERATURE	97	–	–	–	97²				–	
PULSE-RATE	72	72	76	72	76			80	80	
FOETAL HEART-RATE	134	136	136	136	136			138	136	
PAINS { TYPE / FREQUENCY }	–	F 1·10	F 1·5	F 1·5	S 1·3			S 1·3	S 1·2	
URINE PASSED	✓	–	✓	–	✓			✓	✓	
BOWELS OPEN	E.5. Bowel	–	–	–	–			✓	–	

SYMBOLS FOR INDICATING THE TYPE OF PAINS: F—FAIR G—GOOD S—STRONG W—WEAK I—IRREGULAR C—CONTINUOUS

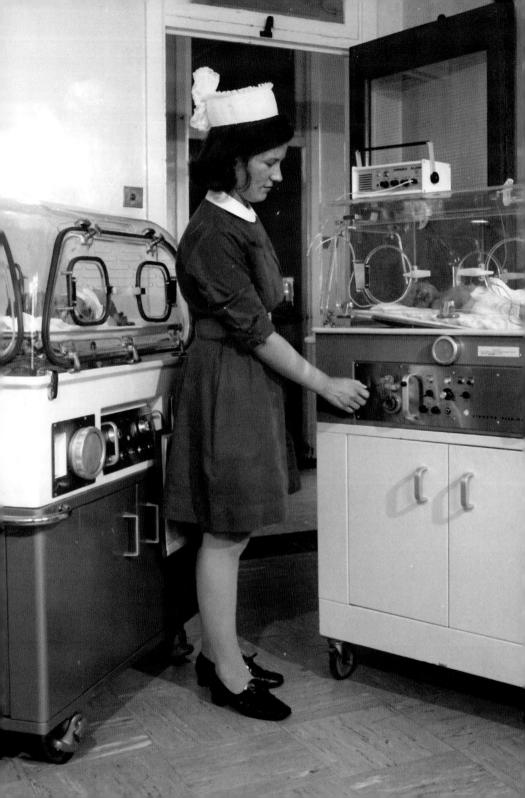

THE 1960s ONWARDS

T HE MIDWIFE'S ROLE changed even more as the move away from home births, encouraged by the NHS, gained momentum in the 1960s. The 1971 Peel Report recommended that every woman give birth in hospital, based largely on the belief that it was a safer environment, and by 1972 the rate of home confinements had dropped to around 8 per cent. Midwifery training was firmly established in hospitals nationwide and in maternity units such as the Edith Watson in Lancashire, which opened in 1968.

Nurse Sheena Byrom embarked on her intensive twelve-month course there in May 1977 and recalled the thrill of getting her uniform, and the prospect of exchanging the white belt for a blue one after six months, identifying her as a senior student. Along with students from Malaysia, the Seychelles and India, she was soon presented with the traditional case book in which she, like her predecessors, had to log all the details of births witnessed – in this case twenty – and babies delivered – forty was the target – during the year. But she nearly missed watching her very first delivery, for at a crucial moment her legs began to wobble and her face felt hot and flushed as the dreaded feeling of clamminess crept up her chest. Fearful of fainting, she rushed out of the room and sat in the cool corridor for half an hour to recover, feeling utterly dismayed. There was some reassurance in being told, by a senior midwife, that her reaction was not unusual, but not all her superiors were as kind, and she

Opposite: These Vickers Medical incubators, about 1970–80, provided a controlled environment for premature babies. They maintained temperature, humidity and oxygen at uniform levels and within fine limits. The 'four-nine' model is on the left, the 'five nine' on the right.

A hospital maternity ward in the 1950s or 1960s.

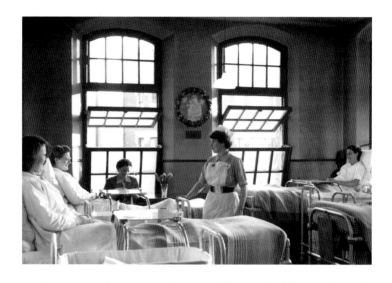

A newborn baby being introduced to his sisters by the midwife, c. 1950s.

was in awe, and even feared some of them. As Sheena learned, there was a strict protocol to be followed when conducting a delivery, beginning with preparing a mother on admission, to opening a sterilised delivery pack and to instructing a mother when to push. Antenatal and postnatal work were all part of district training, and these included weekly checks on mothers and babies in their homes. The conditions of some of these came as a total shock to Sheena, who, unlike her predecessors

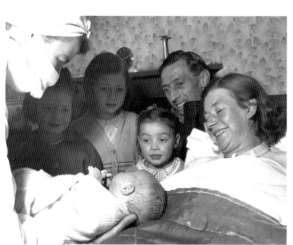

fifty years earlier, had never encountered dire poverty before, but she also revelled in caring for women from the local Pakistani and Indian communities. Like most midwives, her workload vacillated between desperately quiet or rushed off her feet, and being alone on duty at night was not unusual. Having two women in

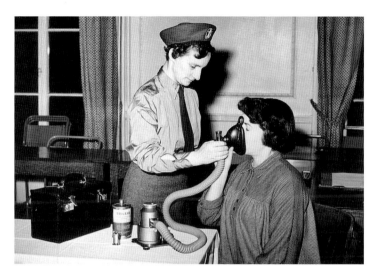

A mother being instructed how to use breathing apparatus during an antenatal visit.

labour at the same time was especially nerve-wracking, and she recalled dashing between their rooms, reassuring each of them and their partners, as she kept hoping they would not deliver simultaneously.

Once they became senior students pupil midwives were allowed to deliver babies unsupervised, but there was always an experienced midwife observing, discreetly hidden behind the glass-panelled door. Student Ros Bradbury learnt an important lesson from one hair-raising situation, when a newborn baby she had delivered failed to cry and needed oxygen: the midwife had to look and sound cool, calm and collected, no matter how panic-stricken she felt inside.

The mothers and children of Deptford waving goodbye to Elsie Walkerdine on her retirement in 1957. She worked as an independent midwife until 1937, and after that (until retirement) for the London County Council.

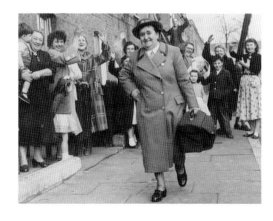

Technology was easing its way into midwifery and by the 1970s adverts began to appear in the *Midwives Chronicle* for fetal monitoring machines. For some in the profession, this was a clear sign that the midwife would no longer need to know how to

Cover from a midwife's drugs book of 1963, in which the use of pethidine for pain relief was recorded.

auscultate (listen to the fetal heart) with a fetal stethoscope. There was less objection to suggestions, put forward in 1963, that domiciliary midwives should be supplied with mobile oxygen apparatus or be provided with car-radio systems so they could get hold of a doctor more easily. The introduction of ultrasound equipment was welcomed as it enabled midwives to view the fetus and estimate gestational age, and it soon became evident that an advanced diploma course was needed to keep midwives up-to-date with these developments.

Pupil midwives soon found that family planning was a standard part of training, but it was the admittance of men onto midwifery courses in the late 1970s that raised some eyebrows. The Sex Discrimination Act, 1975, effectively removed the legal ban on men practising as midwives, and instead introduced transitional arrangements which restricted their entry into the profession. Male midwives got a mixed reception from their female counterparts, with one woman, P. Banks, an SRN and SCM in Wales, writing to the *Midwives Chronicle* in January 1975, expressing her fear that male midwives would be sexually aroused by the sight of the 'exposed female body', and her horror that they would undertake 'intimate nursing duties'. T. Blenkin, a district

THE 1960s ONWARDS　53

midwife in Yorkshire, thought these objections were 'grossly overcharged' and reminded readers that, in accordance with CMB rules, a chaperone could be provided. Women were always asked if they were happy to have a male midwife, and Bryan Beilby, who completed his obstetric nurse training in Brighton in 1977, found he was welcomed unreservedly within the maternity setup.

Domiciliary midwives found themselves called upon to work in GP-led units like the one opened in Oxford in 1966, but this move made Chloe Fisher, who had qualified in 1956, very concerned, for she feared it would prevent her offering mothers the continuity of care she prided herself on. In the end she 'gave in and continued to function there because I had no other choice.' For Sheena Byrom, her time working at Bramley Meade, Whalley, a small, twenty-bed GP-led birthing unit housed in a wealthy mill-owner's converted mansion, was recalled with great affection. Here the midwives treated the mothers like queens, giving them wonderful personal attention. The senior midwife in charge, Carla Gazzola, was on night-duty full time, and was as kind to her staff as she was to the mothers. The prevailing practice was for babies to be taken to the nursery at night, which Sheena recalled occasionally resulted in some mix-ups the next morning. She experienced a moment of sheer panic when a mother politely said 'The baby I gave you last night had a blue name band and this baby has a pink one', but the correct baby was soon located.

The increased use of interventionist monitoring and techniques in hospital deliveries concerned some midwives, including Kay, who was interviewed as part of a survey of consultant obstetric-led units in 1989–90: 'At St Thomas' [London] ... the consultants would routinely induce people when it suited them ... and I thought that was all wrong ... I thought it was ... more natural the way they did things at the smaller hospitals [where] the midwives were ... skilled in normal deliveries without using episiotomies routinely.

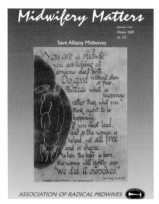
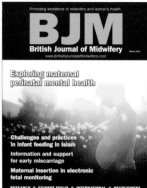
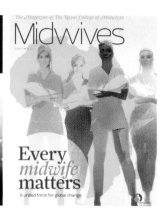

At the Royal Bucks [Buckinghamshire] it wasn't very good. The doctors sort of interfered unnecessarily and if a labour wasn't going as fast as they'd like they'd stick a drip [in] … to speed things along.'

Two student midwives were so troubled by the increasing medicalisation and intervention in NHS maternity care that in 1976 they decided to set up an informal support group for midwives. Their organisation, the Association of Radical Midwives, put the continuity of care and a woman's choice at the heart of their objectives. There were also a small number of women who had chosen to work outside of the NHS, and in July 1985 a group of them got together and formed the Independent Midwives Association. The initial intention was to provide a way of sharing information, but the number of members soon reached double figures and phone enquiries from women interested in engaging a midwife increased, and Independent Midwives UK was established.

Making the decision to leave the NHS and become an independent midwife was a challenging undertaking, as Virginia Howes found out in early 2000. It meant giving up the security of a regular wage, as well as sick and holiday pay and professional indemnity, and she faced erratic and unpredictable working hours as the sole carer of her pregnant client. But for her the opportunity to provide a woman with individualised continuity of care, from the moment she was employed by her until six weeks after the baby was delivered, outweighed the disadvantages.

For decades, midwives had recognised the relaxing benefits of immersion in water during labour as a way of relieving pain, but it was not until the 1980s and 1990s that interest in water births grew in the UK. The maternity unit at Blackpool Victoria Hospital was regularly using birthing pools when Sheena Byrom was asked by Helen, a mother-to-be, to assist in delivering her baby this way, but at home. The prospect was both daunting and exciting, and proved to be an amazing experience for both Sheena and Helen. By the time the Department of Health's landmark report, *Changing Childbirth*, was published in 1993, 96 per cent of births were conducted in hospital. The report identified choice, control and continuity of carer for the mother as the most important tenets of maternity care, but this remains unfinished business. According to the RCM, midwives are still frustrated by the increased medicalisation and standardisation of maternity care, centralisation and the management of NHS maternity services. There is also concern that young midwives and obstetricians are not consulted on how to develop maternity services in future.

Opposite left: The Association of Radical Midwives began by issuing a quarterly newsletter, which evolved into a highly respected journal, *Midwifery Matters*.

Opposite middle: The monthly *British Journal of Midwifery*, launched in 1993, is written by midwives for midwives and aims to keep them up-to-date with the latest developments taking place in clinical midwifery practice.

Opposite right: *Midwives*, the official magazine of the Royal College of Midwives, is published bimonthly. It has appeared under this name since 2008.

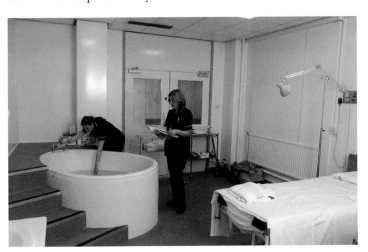

Two midwives prepare a birthing pool, 2003.

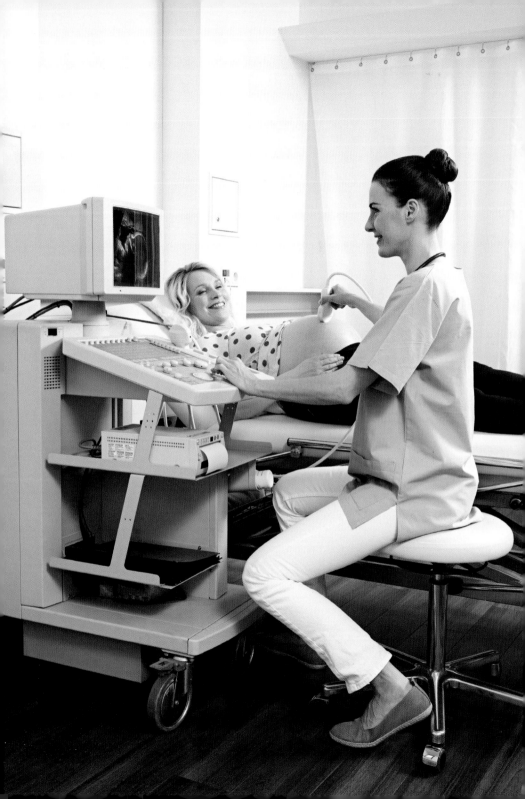

THE TWENTY-FIRST CENTURY

THE TRAINING TO be a midwife in the early twenty-first century has come a long way since the passing of the Midwives Act in 1902. It is now a career that is open to men and women, single or married, and those qualifying are awarded a professional and academic qualification gained through integrated study of theory and practice. The former includes the teaching of management and leadership skills and of effective collaborative practice, as well as research and evidence and how to be a good educator. Supervised practice accounts for half of the programme, with placements on antenatal, labour and postnatal wards, in neonatal units, in

Opposite: A midwife showing an expectant mother ultrasound images.

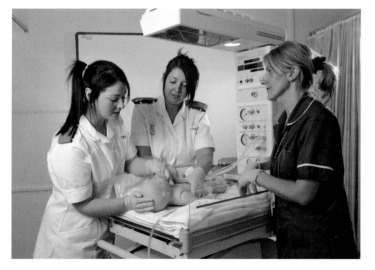

Third-year student midwives being talked through the basic steps of neonatal resuscitation by midwifery lecturer Catriona Jones, as part of the midwifery programme's Complicated Childbirth module at the University of Hull, 2013.

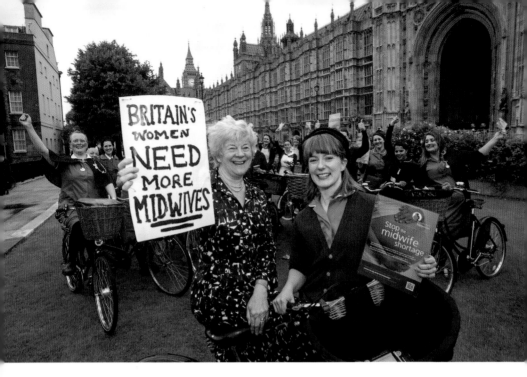

In 2012, mother and newborn baby charity Baby Lifeline in Coventry backed calls for the NHS to recruit 5,000 more midwives, and supported an RCM petition urging the government to recruit and train more specialists. The Care Quality Commission, a national watchdog, had warned that a shortage of midwives was emerging as a problem for NHS trusts.

theatre recovery and within the community. Students are taught how to manage caseloads, gain ward-management experience and develop clinical skills to support and care for women whose pregnancy, labour or postnatal period is not normal or is complicated.

In 2014 there were more than 35,000 qualified midwives on the Nursing and Midwifery Council register, including 197 male midwives, with Sam, the youngest, aged twenty-one. Highly experienced registered midwives, with expertise in a specific field of health care can become consultant midwives, and besides still spending at least half their time working directly with mothers, are involved in research and evaluation, as well as contributing to education, training and development. For Jamie Richardson, working at Whipps Cross University Hospital NHS Trust, this included opening a five-room in-hospital birth centre in May 2006, which aimed to deliver 300 babies a year.

The RCM continues to be the voice of midwifery, and is the UK's only professional organisation and trade union led by midwives, for midwives. The basic starting salary within the NHS in 2015 was £21,692, a far cry from a century earlier, but pay increases continue to be under threat, resulting in unprecedented industrial action by RCM members.

With the exception of about 170 independent midwives, and those who practise in private maternity hospitals, the majority of midwives work within the NHS. Midwives continue to provide advice, care and support for women and their babies during pregnancy, labour and for up to twenty-eight days after the baby has been born. The tools that midwives have at their disposal are the most sophisticated available, but like her predecessors, the midwife must be able to detect problems and call medical help if needed, and be trained in emergency procedures herself. She also has a role in health education and preparation for parenthood, such as teaching antenatal classes. For midwives like Anne W, specialist training in fetal medicine enabled her to

In 2014, Chesterfield Royal Hospital introduced a new IT system allowing all maternity patient records to be kept digitally, enabling more accurate note-keeping and more effective care, tailored for every patient.

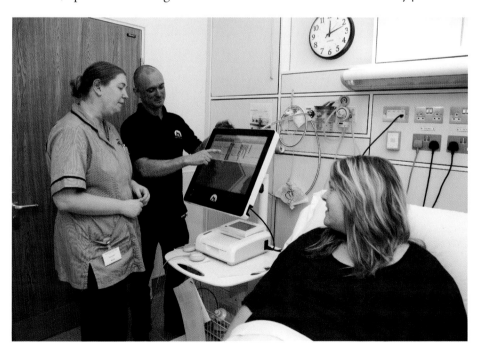

In hospital, a mother learning to bathe her newborn baby with help from the father and a midwife.

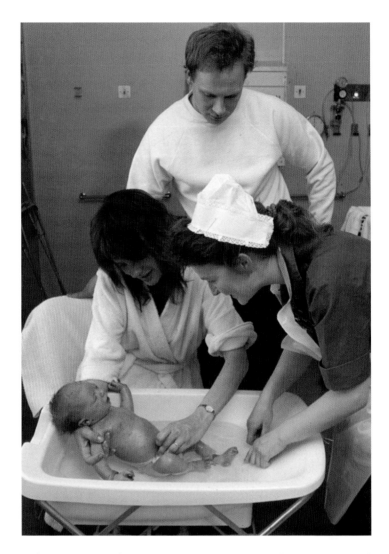

offer parents professional care, support and advice during and after challenging pregnancies.

Within the community, midwives mostly work as part of a team, for example within GP surgeries and health centres, and are able to offer a degree of continuity of care. Unlike a century ago, the opportunity to attend births at home is rare, for the vast majority of babies are delivered in a hospital environment, either on labour wards or in midwife-led birthing units. New birth centres such as the one opened in Blackburn, East Lancashire in late 2010, aim to offer one-to-one care from community midwives, as well as home births. For Margaret Wilson, a local retired community midwife, this move was a positive one, a return to the earlier maternity homes where she had worked, and a step towards making birth 'a normal process again' in a supportive and stress-free environment. Medical advances have transformed the range of diagnostic and palliative support that the midwife has at her disposal, and these are reflected in highly reduced infant and maternal mortality rates. In 2013 there were just 3.8 deaths per 1,000 live births, compared with 130 deaths for every 1,000 children born in 1911.

Midwifery remains a stressful and exhausting job, the hours are long with day and night shifts and on-call rotas, and many midwives struggle to balance their professional and family lives. But as Maria Anderson concluded in her 2012 book, *Tales of a Midwife*, 'midwifery is not a job; it is a way of life. You have to give a lot of yourself and make it your world. And when you do, you can make a real difference.'

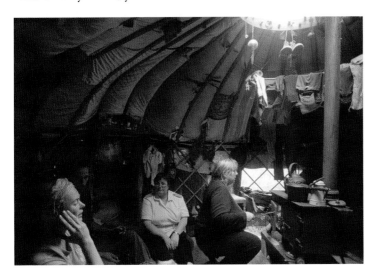

A midwife, seated on floor cushions, visiting two pregnant women in 2000 in the living quarters of a rural Scottish commune, where the women planned to give birth.

FURTHER READING

Browne, Alan (ed.). *Masters, Midwives, and Ladies-in-Waiting: Rotunda Hospital, 1745–1995*. A. & A. Farmar, 1995.

Byrom, Sheena. *Catching Babies: A Midwife's Tale*. Headline, 2011.

Cowell, Betty and Wainwright, David. *Behind the Blue Door. The History of the Royal College of Midwives 1881–1981*. Cassell Ltd, 1981.

Donnison, Jean. *Midwives and Medical Men. A History of the Struggle for the Control of Childbirth*. Historical Publications, 1988.

Dunn, Dot May. *Twelve Babies on a Bike: Diary of a Pupil Midwife*. Orion, 2010.

Howes, Virginia. *The Baby's Coming: A Story of Dedication by an Independent Midwife*. Headline, 2014.

Loudon, Irvine. *The Tragedy of Childbed Fever*. Oxford University Press, 2000.

Reid, Lindsay. *Scottish Midwives: Twentieth-Century Voices*, 2nd ed. Black Devon Books, 2008.

Williams, A. Susan. *Women and Childbirth in the Twentieth Century. History of the National Birthday Trust Fund 1928–93*. Sutton Press, 1997.

Worth, Jennifer. *Call The Midwife*, Weidenfeld & Nicolson, 2012.

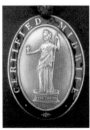

Below: A State Certified Midwife badge.

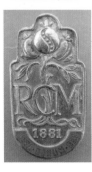

Bottom: The new Royal College of Midwives badge. The College of Midwives was granted its Royal Charter in June 1947, becoming the Royal College of Midwives.

The Library of the Royal College of Obstetricians and Gynaecologists contains the Royal College of Midwives' archives and displays artefacts.

RCOG, 27 Sussex Place, Regent's Park, London NW1 4RG. Telephone: 020 7772 6200

Website: www.rcog.org.uk/en/guidelines-research-services/ library-services/archives-and-heritage

UK Centre for the History of Nursing and Midwifery www.nursing.manchester.ac.uk/ukchnm

ACKNOWLEDGMENTS

ROYAL COLLEGE OF MIDWIVES (RCM)

Images taken from *Nursing Notes/Midwives Chronicle*: July 1906 (p.101), page 14; May 1914 (p.143), page 16; November 1923 (xiii), page 21; March 1925 (p.1), page 24; March 1935 (p.49), page 32; November 1946 (pp.222–3), page 42, and all reproduced by kind permission of the RCM.

From the Papers of Edith Pye, RCMS/2, pages 11 (bottom), 15; and from the Papers of Mrs Fagan, RCMS/42, both held in the archives of the RCM and reproduced by kind permission of the RCM.

Photographs held in the archives of the RCM

RCM/PH7/2/15, page 3; RCMS/144, page 13; RCM/PH/7/1/2, © of Chris Wade, Photographer of Keystone Press Agency, London EC4, page 29; RCM/PH7/5/7, page 31; RCM/PH7/2/12, © of Ellis Sykes, Photographer, 165 Brompton Road SW5, page 42; RCM/PH7/2/10, page 43; RCM/PH7/2/5, © RCM, page 44; RCM/PH7/2/61(top), © RCM, page 45; RCM/PH7/2/78 (bottom), © RCM page 45; RCM/PM7/2/19, page 46; RCMS/21, page 47; RCM/PH7/2/30, © Vickers Ltd, Millbank Tower, Millbank, London SW1, page 49; RCM/PH7/2/6 (top), page 50; RCM/PH7/2/59 (bottom), page 50; RCM/176, page 52. All these have been reproduced by kind permission of the RCM .

IMAGES FROM OTHER SOURCES

Association of Radical Midwives/ Sarah Montagu calligraphy, page 54 (left); Sally Bosley, page 23 (centre); Chesterfield Royal Hospital NHS Foundation Trust, page 59; Faculty of Health and Social Care, Midwifery Programme, University of Hull, page 57; Getty Images/ Joos Mind, page 56; Judy Godby/Brocket's Babies, page 38; Rob Higgins, page 20; Mrs Elizabeth Longman, page 18; Long Whatton History Society, page 34 (bottom); Peter Maleczek, page 63 (right); MA Healthcare, page 54 (middle); Helen Owen, page 36; Queen's Nursing Institute, pages 12, 41; RCM: Papers of Edith Pye, pages 11 (bottom), 15; Royal College of Midwives: Nicholas Hallam, page 58; Barnet Saidman/Queen's Nursing Institute, page 43 (bottom); Salvation Army, page 17; Science and Society Picture Library, page 51 (bottom); Terrence Ross/Long Whatton History Society, page 39 (bottom); Topfoto, front cover; Wellcome Images/Science Museum, London, page 7; Wellcome Images/L.Durrell McKenna, page 61; Wellcome Images/Anthea Sieveking, page 60; Wellcome Library, pages 1, 4 , 6 (both), 8, 9 , 10 (bottom),11 (top), 13, 17 (bottom), 20 (bottom), 25, 27 (bottom), 34, 51 (top), 55 (bottom), 60; Carolyn Wilding, pages 26, 30; Eric Wilkinson/Schools of Nursing, page 23 (right); Stuart Williams, page 8 (bottom); Keith Wright, page 22.

INDEX